What You Should Know About HPV

<u>INTRODUCTION</u>

HPV is a combination of viruses that may cause warts on the genitals, hands or feet.

Some HPV's may cause cervical cancer.

A HPV vaccination may protect you from the virus and it is now available to the public.

At least 50% of the population contract HPV in their lifetime.

Most people do not have any symptoms from the HPV and it goes away on its own.

Some HPV's do cause cervical cancer as well as cancer of the anus and the male penis.

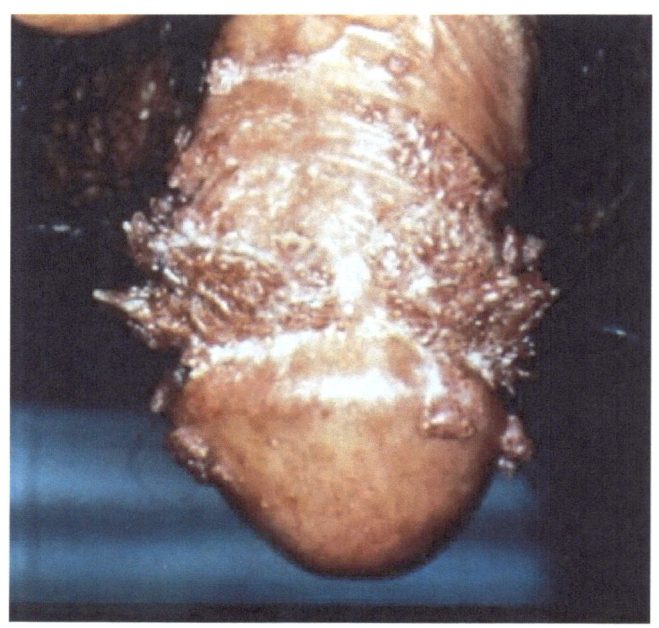

Genital Warts of a Male Penis

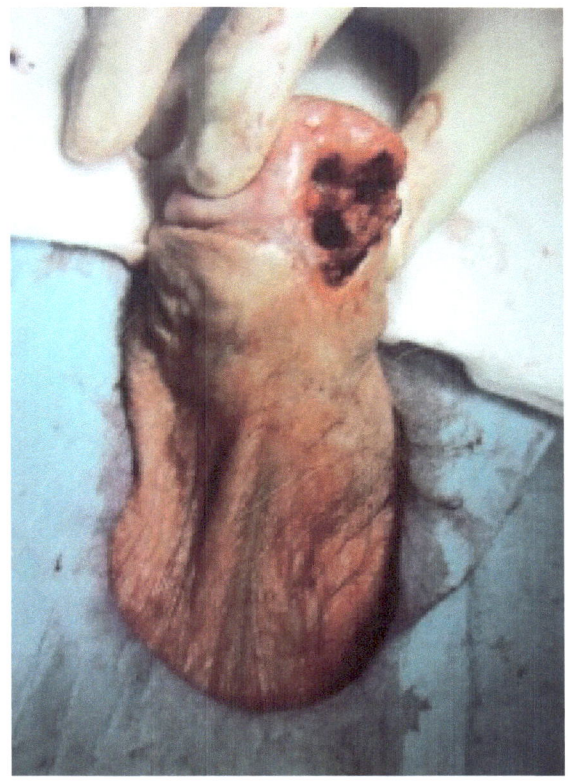

Penis cancer from HPV

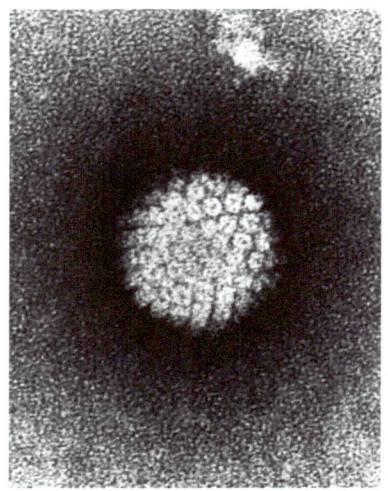

HPV virus

HPV FACTS

There are about 100 HPV viruses today.

Each one is named by type or given a number.

The type or number is assigned by the type of wart that results from the type of wart that the individual may have contracted.

HPV stands for Human Papillomavirus.

The HPV virus is found in the body's epithelial cells.

This is where the virus lives and dwells.

The HPV cells are thin and flat cells that can be found of the skin's surface and in or around moist areas such as the cervix, anus, mouth, throat, penis head, vagina or vulva.

There are 100 HPV viruses.

About 60% cause the warts on the hands and feet.

The other 40% are sexually transmitted.

The 40% are drawn to moist areas such as a person's genital region or their anus.

THE SPREADING OF HPV

The HPV virus is spread through sexual contact with an infected partner.

The moist genital area is exposed most often and sometimes using a condom does not protect the individual if the other sexual partner has been exposed to the virus.

Some partners may not know that they are actually infected with the HPV virus. You must remember that they may have no signs of contracting the sexually transmitted disease.

HPV IS VERY COMMON

The CDC reports that approximately 20 million people are exposed to the HPV virus in their lifetime.

About ¾ of people between the ages of 15-49 will be exposed to this virus within their lifetime.

A person is more apt to get HPV if they have:

➢ **Multiple sexual partners**
➢ **Have sex with a partner that has had multiple sexual partners**
➢ **Have sex at an early age**

**The CDC reports that HPV can affect anyone.
The statistics show the following:**

➢ **45% of women of the ages between 14-19 were exposed to the HPV virus**
➢ **27% of women of the ages of 20-24 were exposed to the HPV virus**
➢ **19% of women between the ages of 50-59 have been exposed to the HPV virus**

PEOPLE MAY WONDER WHAT HAPPENS AFTER THEY ARE EXPOSED TO HPV

Most people never know that they are even exposed to HPV.
90% of all women never know that they have been exposed.
The human body actually gets rid of the virus after about two years.
HPV can cause changes in the cervix of women and it could also cause changes in the penile tissue or the anus.

HOW CAN A PERSON DECREASE THEIR CHANCES OF GETTING HPV

To be perfectly frank, the only way to avoid the chance of getting exposed to HPV is to not have sex at all.

This also includes ORAL SEX.

Another way is to avoid having multiple sexual partners.

Another way is to try and get the HPV vaccine.

You must also know that some people have the HPV virus and they never even know it at all.

<u>SYMPTOMS OF HPV</u>

Some people may not show any symptoms at all. Therefore, they may not know that they transfer the virus.
Other people may have warts appear on their genital region.
The warts can appear on or in the vagina, cervix, vulva or penis.
These warts can cause abnormal cervical cells or abnormal anus cells.
It depends on what type that the individual may contract from an infected partner.

SOME TREATMENTS FOR HPV

Some treatments of HPV may include but not limited to:

➢ **Cryotherapy**

➢ **Surgical Removal**

➢ **Electro-cautery**

➢ **Applying a topical acid**

➢ **Laser vaporization**

<u>CONCLUSIONS</u>

If you or someone you know has been exposed to the HPV virus, you need to seek medical attention and advice.
This may prevent further outbreaks in the future.

The End

This self-help book about HPV was written to help people who may think that they have been exposed to this sexually transmitted disease. Sometimes it is undetected and people may never know that they have contracted it. The body usually gets rid of the virus in about two years but the virus may come back also because it lies dormant in your epithelial tissues. So, if you or someone you know thinks that they have been exposed to this virus, please seek medical attention and advice as soon as possible.

Misty Lynn Wesley has a diversified career portfolio in the medical, legal, fashion and insurance industries. She is an avid blogger for Examiner.com, Helium, and Yahoo Voices. She also writes for CBS Local out of St. Paul, MN sometimes and Believe.com. She has written four books with Publish America and several on Amazon.com. She and her chosen producers have produced several audio books on Amazon, Barnes and Noble and I tunes. Check them out if you have time. God bless.

www.ingramcontent.com/pod-product-compliance
Lightning Source LLC
Chambersburg PA
CBHW050926290526
45792CB00002B/898